# Ketogenic Diet:

*Low-Carb, High Fat Diet Done Properly For Real Weight Loss!*

*2nd Edition*

# Contents

# Introduction

Thank you for choosing this book "Ketogenic Diet: Low-Carb, High Fat Diet Done Properly For Real Weight Loss!"

In this book you will learn everything that you need to know about the Ketogenic diet and the lifestyle changes that you can adapt to achieve your weight and fitness goals. This isn't one of those glossy books that promise weight reduction within no time. It will take some serious time and commitment from you to actually make any difference. So, be prepared to make a few changes if you really want this diet to be of any use.

The concept of Ketogenic diet is quite simple. This is a low-carb and a high fat diet. When this diet is followed properly, you will be pleasantly surprised. So, resist your temptations, put in some effort and give this book a thorough reading to lead a happier and a much healthier life. Happy reading!

# Chapter 1: All About the Ketogenic Diet

A Ketogenic diet is a low carbohydrate diet where the ketones that are produced by the liver are used as a source of energy. It is also known as the Keto diet or the low-carb and high fat diet. Whenever we consume food that contains carbohydrates, it is immediately converted into glucose and insulin by our body. Glucose is a molecule that is readily converted into energy hence it is chosen over other sources. Meanwhile, insulin is produced by our body to process the glucose present in the blood stream. Since our body is using up all the glucose, it becomes the primary source of energy while fats is just stored up. An average person's diet is high in carbohydrates which implies that the main source of energy is glucose.

When there is a reduction in the intake of carbs, the body is induced into ketosis. Ketosis occurs naturally when the intake of food is low to aid in our survival. In this state, the body produces ketones and are used as a source of energy.

The general idea of the Ketogenic diet is to force the body into a state of ketosis. This is achieved by reducing the intake of carbohydrates and not just by starving the body of calories. Furthermore, when there is an increase in the intake of fats and decrease in the carbs consumed, the body starts burning up the ketones to maintain the required level of energy.

## Fast facts about the Ketogenic diet

The following are the facts that you need to know to get a better understanding of this diet:

### It is designed to induce a state of ketosis.

Like the name suggests, this diet is designed to induce the body into a state of ketosis by reducing the consumption of carbohydrates.

Primarily, the body's source of fuel is carbs and the main source of energy is the easily convertible glucose. When the supply of glucose is restricted, the body moves towards making use of another source of energy which is fat. A normal Ketogenic diet would consist of 70% fats, 20% of proteins and about 5% of carbs.

## *The primary source of fuel is fat*

What we consume, be it fats or carbohydrates, are metabolized and stored by the body. Carbohydrates are broken down into glucose and stored in the muscles and liver, whereas fats are broken down into triglycerides and stored as adipose tissues or body fat. Glucose and triglycerides are both sources of energy. In keto diet, as the body is in ketosis, the fats will be the primary source of fuel and energy. Of course, there is still a need to consume protein.

## *Low carbs signify low energy*

Reducing the intake of carbs will not help you with your exercise regime. When the store of glucose in the body is gradually depleted, it becomes increasingly difficult to exercise. This is why all the endurance sports require the athletes to consume energy drinks and other substitutes. In following the ketogenic diet, the depleted glucose is replaced by ketones and gradually gets the body to get used to burning fat efficiently.

## *Watch out for high cholesterol*

In keto diet, the body starts burning fat to generate energy. Consequently, you might end up with high cholesterol. Cholesterol, a fatty substance, is naturally produced in the body and also found in the food we eat. The increased consumption of foods with LDL cholesterol or bad cholesterol clogs the arteries and causes heart diseases. To counter this, lots of fiber and good fats are highly recommended.

### *Read food labels and pay attention to the nutrient content*

The keto diet requires carb consumption of 50 grams per day or less. In order to achieve this, you will have to start reading the food labels carefully. Most dairy products are high in protein as well as carbohydrates. This also applies to some of the fruits, nuts, legumes and even vegetables. Be wise in your food choices as you commit yourself to this diet.

### Carbohydrate cheats

This diet is a real challenge because all the food we eat on a daily basis is mostly made of carbohydrates. Spaghetti Bolognese will not be the same without the spaghetti, right? This is where carbohydrate cheats come in. You need to find low-carb alternatives like replacing rice with cauliflower rice or zucchini ribbons instead of pasta. Almond flour and peanut flour are healthy as well. Consider this, a portion of 1/4th cup of cooked brown rice or even one boiled sweet potato consists of almost as much as 12.5 grams of carbs. Research each food's carbohydrate content and compare them as you go along this diet.

## Side effects to look out for

Aside from the desired effect of losing weight, there are also some side effects to be aware of in the keto diet. These are nausea, headache, lethargy and sleepiness. This diet can be tough on both the body and the mind. Some people have had cognitive reduction (fogginess, increased confusion etc.) and mood swings. A combination of these symptoms is referred to as the Keto flu. These side effects are on a case to case basis and not the same for everyone. However, it is best to seek professional advice or consult your dietician before and during the diet for some healthy guidelines.

## Nutritional deficits must be addressed effectively

The diet would make your body get rid of sodium, potassium and water content drastically resulting to the Keto flu. While the body is capable of adjusting to any minor changes in the level of electrolytes, an increase in the water intake will cause an imbalance in the electrolytes. Water is good but we do not want to spoil the harmony of electrolytes in the body. Also, steer clear of sweetened drinks.

## Bad breath

This diet will definitely give you a bad breath. Ketones are produced when fat is burned for energy instead of carbohydrates. The ketones provide energy to the brain. With all that burning of excessive fat, the amount of ketones produced is also high. One way the body gets rid of excess ketones is through breath, hence the bad breath. Since the root cause of this problem isn't deficiency in oral health, you can't get rid of this problem by brushing or flossing. The only practical way to get rid of it is by consuming more carbs which will be in contradictory with what the keto diet promotes. A temporary solution would be breath mints.

# Chapter 2: Myths About Fat Consumption

Fats aren't that bad. In fact, consumption of fats is good for your body. It is the mindset towards fat that has given it a bad reputation. In this chapter we will take a look at some myths about consumption of fats that have caused unnecessary fear.

## Myth#1 - Consumption of fat will make you fat.

This isn't true. The fat in our ordinary diet is different from the one that is stored in our body. The body takes a lot more time to digest fat than any other nutrient source and the feeling of fullness comes from the nutrients. Technically, the consumption of fat would help cut down on calorie intake which is actually good. Fat is a nutrient just like proteins and carbohydrates. It helps in the absorption of vitamins and when broken down into fatty acids it also sustains the brain. So consumption of fats is quintessential for your good health.

Still, eating fatty foods must be in moderation. Eating too much of it together with refined carbohydrates can lead to unnecessary weight gain.

## Myth#2 - There are healthy and unhealthy fats.

It is a general misconception that fats are only of two kinds: the good ones and the bad ones where trans fat and saturated fats are the bad fats while unsaturated ones are good. Well, the distinction between these fats is more complicated. Fats are of seven kinds. The type of fats ranging from the most to the least healthy are: Omega 3 fats, monounsaturated fats, polyunsaturated fats, saturated fats, medium chain triglycerides, Omega 6 fatty acids and then Trans fat. What you should focus on is eating fats that fall in the top of the above mentioned list.

# Myth#3 - Trans fat isn't all that bad.

Even small amounts of trans fat will shorten our life span because they get accumulated in the body. Bacteria are incapable of digesting trans fats thus it is added to some processed foods to increase its shelf life. Whenever you consume trans fat, the body does not digest it so it ends up lining and clogging the body's arteries and liver. As a result, there is an increased risk of developing various coronary diseases, cardio vascular diseases as well as damage to arteries.

# Myth#4- Foods labeled with 0 grams trans fat are perfectly safe.

Avoiding trans fat at any cost is a must in this diet. While buying food products, do pay some heed to their labels. If per serving a product contains less than 0.4 grams of trans fat, then it legally can be listed as 0 grams trans fat. Let's say you bought it and end up consuming four servings of such food products. Computing that, your consumption of trans fat is 2 grams. This might not seem much, but it can definitely make you sick. A really effective way to detect foods that contain trans fat is by reading their labels carefully. *Partially hydrogenated oil* in the ingredients used also contains trans fat, avoid it as well.

# Myth#5- For better health, consume less saturated fats.

For years, we have been blaming saturated fats for all the cardiovascular diseases. In truth, saturated fats are cardiovascular neutral meaning they neither cause nor help these diseases. People who consume a lot meats and food rich in saturated fats are at a higher risk when compared to those who don't or eat less of such foods. Still, the same can be said if the saturated fats are replaced with processed and refined carbs with added sugars in a person's diet. Even if you avoid greasy bacon for breakfast and eat sugary cereal, the risk of heart diseases is the same. A diet that is full of refined carbs is as bad as a diet full of saturated fats from meats and various other sources. It's still a matter of making healthy food choices.

## Myth#6- Full fat dairy products are bad for the health.

The fat in dairy products is absorbed differently from the fats in other foods. People who consume full fat dairy products in fact are less likely to be overweight than others who do not consume the same. Their risk to high blood pressure and type-2 diabetes is significantly lower and more likely to live longer compared to those who consume the low fat dairy varieties.

## Myth#7 - The healthiest of oils is olive oil.

Olive oil indeed is very healthy. Unfortunately, when heated up, its healthy monounsaturated fats are converted into saturated fats and even to trans fat. Going back to myth #2, these fats are at the bottom of the healthy list. Healthier alternatives are peanut oil, avocado and sesame oils.

## Myth#8- Salad dressings are unhealthy

Dietary fiber is very important to the body. It is required in absorbing the nutrients in the food. Completely avoiding fat in salad dressings is no good. In forgoing the dressings or making use of fat free dressing like vinegar, you might be cutting on the calories but it really won't do your body any good.

## Myth#9- Cardio can burn fat.

There's a grain of truth in this statement but this does not happen immediately. There's around 1000 calories stored in the liver that are easy to burn. This reserve needs to be burned out before the body can start breaking down fat for fuel. Even an hour of cardio does not burn 1000 calories. Don't worry about how to burn through the calorie store in your body, every little amount of exercise you do will bring you a step closer to achieving your goal.

# Chapter 3: Benefits of Ketogenic Diet

Health professionals demonize diets that are low in carb and high in fat content across the world. It was a popular belief that such diets would exponentially increase the chances of individuals of beings susceptible to heart diseases, all due to the high content of fat. Well, this isn't the case these days. Since the beginning of this century a lot of research has been conducted and most of the results point out that keto diets are much better when compared to the others. A low-carb diet not only helps in shedding weight but it also helps in improving the overall health and correcting major health risks like cholesterol. Let us take a look at ten benefits of the Ketogenic diet:

## Reduction in appetite (not in a bad way)

The most difficult side effect to cope with while dieting is hunger. This is the most leading reason why a lot of people give up on their diets. An advantage of a low-carb diet is it aids in the reduction of your appetite. Once you start cutting down on carbohydrate intake and replacing it with protein and fat, the amount of calories you consume will also be reduced. The decrease in carbs intake in turn decreases a person's appetite.

## Facilitates in more weight loss

One of the simplest and the most effective way to shed the extra kilos is by cutting down on carbs. Studies show that a person who is on a low-carb diet when compared to a low fat diet is bound to reduce weight more rapidly. One reason is that the excess water present in the body is removed. Once the insulin level in the body is reduced and the kidneys start getting rid of the sodium, there is a noticeable weight loss in the first week.

The keto diet is observed to be very effective for the first six months or so. It would remain effective if maintained as a lifestyle. Eating low-carb is a diet and a way of life at the same time. In accepting and believing this, the process would be much easier to adjust to. Always find ways to accommodate healthier options for carbohydrates into your diet once you have achieved your ideal weight. It wouldn't be an exaggeration to say that a low-carb diet will definitely help in rapid weight loss, provided you follow it regularly and consistently.

## Abdominal fat will be shed.

All the fat present in the body is not the same. Health risks vary depending upon the location and concentration of fats in the body. They are mostly stored either under our skin as a layer of fat or in the abdominal cavity. Visceral fat tends to accumulate around the organs that may result in inflammation and obstruction of insulin making it one of the prominent causes of metabolism dysfunction.

A low-carb diet is very effective in getting rid of this harmful fat in the viscera and abdominal cavity. Adapting to the Ketogenic lifestyle reduces the risk of heart diseases and even type-2 diabetes over a period of time.

## Reduction of triglycerides

Triglycerides are molecules of fat present in the body from the breaking down of fats. An increase in the amount of triglycerides in the blood likewise increases the risk of heart diseases. This increase of triglycerides is attributed to the consumption of carbohydrates specifically simple sugar fructose. The obvious effect of following a low-carb diet is the reduction in triglycerides levels in the blood. Oppositely, a low-fat diet increases triglycerides levels in the blood.

The amount of triglycerides is directly proportional to the amount of carbs that you consume. Furthermore, the higher the triglyceride, the higher is the risk of heart diseases.

## Improvement in the level of good cholesterol

High-density lipoprotein (HDL) is often referred to as the good cholesterol. Technically, it is incorrect to refer to it as cholesterol since all the cholesterol molecules have the same composition. HDL and LDL are the lipoproteins that help in the transportation of cholesterol in the blood stream.

Low-density lipoprotein (LDL) is responsible for carrying the cholesterol molecules to the liver and the rest of the body whereas the high-density lipoprotein (HDL) is responsible for carrying the cholesterol molecules away from the body, either for reuse or excretion.

A higher level of HDL means that the risk of heart diseases is lower. One of the most efficient ways of increasing HDL is by the consumption of healthy fats. Low-carb diets recommend this as well. It comes as no surprise that the HDL levels of individuals who follow the Ketogenic diet are high when compared to those who follow a low-fat diet. The ratio of triglycerides and LDL is also another indicator of risk for heart diseases. The higher this ratio is the greater is the risk of heart diseases. Reduction in the level of triglycerides and the simultaneous increase in the levels of HDL can be achieved by following a low-carb diet.

## Reduction in the level of both insulin and blood sugar

The carbs that we consume are broken down into simple sugars in the digestive system. Simple sugars enter our blood stream and increase the level of blood sugar. High levels of blood sugars is extremely toxic to the body thus the body produces a hormone called insulin. Insulin helps the cells to bring glucose to the cells either to burn it as energy or store it. Normally, this insulin response is the body's way of reducing a spike in the blood sugar to prevent any further damage to the body.

One of the most common problems plaguing mankind is diabetes. This is a metabolic disease where the pancreas is not producing enough insulin or the body cells are not reacting properly to the insulin present in the blood. One type of this is the type-2 diabetes where the body fails to generate sufficient insulin to help in the breakdown of blood sugars in the blood. A simple solution is to cut down on carbs consumption. There will be no more need to generate more insulin thus, both the blood sugar levels and insulin levels decrease. If you are on medication to reduce your blood sugar and want to follow the Ketogenic diet, consult your doctor first because the dosage of your medication might need to be adjusted for the prevention of hypoglycemia.

To sum it up, reduce the amount of carbs you consume to reduce the blood sugar and insulin levels.

## Lowered blood pressure

Hypertension or having abnormally high levels of blood pressure is a leading factor in causing heart diseases and other diseases like kidney failure and damage to eye sight. The Ketogenic diet will help in controlling the levels of blood pressure and reducing the risk of the above-mentioned diseases.

## Promotes treatment of metabolic syndrome

Metabolic syndrome is a medical condition associated with a high risk of diabetes and heart diseases. Its symptoms are elevated blood pressure and sugar levels, abdominal obesity, high levels of triglycerides and low levels of HDL. These symptoms when not kept in check, will eventually lead to various heart diseases and even type-2 diabetes as well. Successfully fight and reverse all these symptoms by following the Ketogenic diet. Disappointingly, the government as well as key health organizations still recommend a low fat diet when these symptoms can be effectively reversed by following a low-carb diet.

## An improved LDL levels

Low Density Lipoprotein (LDL) carries the cholesterol molecules to the liver and the rest of the body. Research shows that people with high levels of LDL are often more prone to heart diseases. Recent studies show that it is important to identify the type of LDL present in the body because not all of them are equal. To determine the type of LDL, the criteria is based on its size. Individuals who have small particles of LDL are more prone to heart diseases than the ones who have large particles of it. Following a low-carb diet increases the size of the LDL particles while its number floating in the blood stream are reduced.

Keto diet have two positive results on LDL particles: 1. its size increases making them benign and 2. its concentration in the blood stream decreases.

## Helps in treating several disorders of the brain

FACT: The brain needs a constant supply of glucose. A part of the brain is equipped for burning glucose only. This is why our liver produces glucose even out of protein when we don't consume any carbs. Fortunately, a major portion of our brain can burn ketones as well and these are produced either when our body is being starved or when the carb intake has been reduced. This is the mechanism that has been made use of during the Ketogenic diet. It has proven to be effective in treating epilepsy, especially in children who do not respond to any other form of treatment. A study shows that when children suffering from epilepsy were made to follow the Ketogenic diet, there was about 50% decrease in seizures.

Of late, studies on diets based on low or no carbohydrates consumption in correlation to brain disorders like Alzheimer's and Parkinson's are being conducted.

# Chapter 4: Side Effects of Over-consumption of Carbs

A healthy and balanced diet is the key to good health. Overeating creates an imbalance leading to a number of nasty after effects. The calories stored in the body increase exponentially leading to obesity and other problems related to it. Stress eating is a common scenario. We tend to crave carbohydrates in times of stress that later on becomes a bad eating habit. The following are the side effects of consuming too much refined and processed carbohydrates:

## Blood sugar levels imbalance

Like mentioned earlier, too much of anything is not beneficial for the body. Too much refined carbohydrates in particular messes with the blood sugar levels. When you eat a slice of cake with frosting on it, it increases the levels of insulin in the body and results in the storage of glucose. Insulin balances out blood sugar levels and keeps them in a normal range. As blood sugar levels rise, the pancreas secretes more insulin. If the body does not produce enough insulin or the cells are resistant to the effects of insulin, hyperglycemia develops and causes long-term complications when not addressed. These imbalances in the blood stream tend to disrupt the functioning of the human body as a whole.

## Weight gain

Consumption of foods high in saturated fats or even carbs will result in unnecessary weight gain. Foods that are rich in refined carbs lead to weight gain because they are mostly empty calories that lead to more carb craving. There are a couple of healthy sources to get your carbohydrates requirement like fruits and vegetables. So instead of picking a bowl of pasta, opt for your favorite protein. Find alternatives for carbs and stick to those for a healthier life.

# Functioning of the brain

Brain fatigue or brain fog is an episode of mental confusion brought about by many factors, one of which is diabetes. It is characterized by confusion, a lack of focus, poor memory recall, and reduced mental acuity. Fluctuating glucose levels in the blood can cause short term brain fatigue symptoms.

# Chapter 5: Things to Consider

Ketogenic diet is not just a diet but a lifestyle choice. It is not a fad. This diet is backed by research that shows the manner in which the metabolism of our body changes when we cut back on the consumption of carbohydrates and increase the fats consumed. There are certain things that you will have to consider before you get started with this diet and this chapter talks about these in detail.

## Seek professional help

It will be helpful if you can consult a professional or a health care practitioner who can help you chalk out a proper meal plan. It will also help you avoid mistakes along the way and ensure that your body is not deprived of any important macro-nutrients. Getting started on a diet is not really difficult when you know what you are supposed to do and what you can and cannot eat. Figuring out all this on your own might prove to be a challenge. The very idea of going through this tedious process might be a turn off for a lot of people. Individuals who are suffering epilepsy should consider the diet with their nutritionist before they get started with it. Even if you are on any medication, do consult your doctor before giving this diet a go, especially when it comes to children.

## Blood tests are important

Get a complete blood work done before starting on this diet to ensure that you aren't suffering from any condition that you might not be aware of. Consult your physician once you get your results and seek approval to get on with this diet. Some suggested tests to get done are lipid profile, thyroid panel, inflammatory markers, full blood count and tests for liver/kidney functioning. If you suffer from fatigue then you can add a little of B12 supplements to your meal to get rid of anemia.

## There's no rush

Take it easy, especially during the initial stages of this diet. There's no need to cut down your carbohydrate intake straight away. Gradually decrease carbohydrate intake over a period of few weeks. Some doctors even recommend a fast to ensure that your body goes into ketosis easily, but do not do this if you haven't done it before. Consult a doctor first.

## Select the timing

It might not be the most ideal time for the implementation of this diet if you are busy (physically, emotionally or even psychologically) for two reasons. The first one is that you will be stressed about cooking with certain restrictions. Meals and the method of preparation employed will take a little getting used. It will be like setting yourself up for failure when you are off to a shaky start. Second, it will be challenging, not impossible but it will take a toll on you adding more to the stress you are already in.

Let us take the instance of a cancer patient. If the patient has started with chemotherapy, it is not advisable to follow this diet immediately. It will be extremely difficult because most of the drugs used in chemotherapy have a glucose base. This means that the level of glucose in the body will be high and ketosis will be non-existent. It would be helpful instead to finishing chemotherapy, maintaining a good metabolic balance by exercising and eating balanced food rich in nutrients. Take sufficient time to let the body cope with all the medication. For an athlete, select an appropriate time to put this diet into action. It does not make sense to go on a keto diet on competition season as it will mean giving up on carbs and a reduction in the energy produced by the body. The body's adaptation to this lifestyle can range from a week to a month. This is a risk you shouldn't take when the conditions are not favorable.

## Plan ahead

This diet can't be done randomly. Research and read on Ketogenic diets to be equipped on meals and all the necessary requirements.

Plan ahead, make a list, and get some grocery shopping done. Depending upon your body type, there will also be some foods that might not provide you sufficient nourishment. You will also need to make a list of things you might be allergic to. Take into consideration some food sensitivity symptoms connected to consumption of some food products like an increased heart rate after a meal, constipation, mood swings and other digestive problems. One good thing about following the Ketogenic diet is that most of the products that are likely to cause allergic reactions like wheat or even peanuts are mostly eliminated. Only when you have a better idea of what all you can consume without having to face any unpleasantness will you be able to achieve the optimal results from this diet.

## Social life

Once you start this diet, commit to follow it to see some substantial improvement. This means that you will have to stick to your diet even while eating out, socializing and travelling as well. This might be a little difficult in the beginning. You don't want your diet to clash with any major events that are coming up in your life like a birthday party or even a vacation. A little bit of planning and mental toughening is required. A lot of people might comment about the foods that you consume. Be ready for a verbal onslaught of gasps and sighs. It is normal that people would comment when they see you gorging on fat and protein while ignoring the carbs. Ignore all the advice you get from others apart from the one given to you by your doctor.

## Essentials

Ketone or glucose meters and even weighing scales are essentials aside from the food. Weigh out your foods before you consume them. This extra effort will go a long way for the diet to work properly. Some kitchen equipment like a good blender, steamer, non-toxic fry pans, and proper storage containers when you want to freeze any of the food cooked are also recommended to be on hand.

## Keep going, don't give up

You will need to keep going even after achieving the optimal state of ketosis. One way in which you can do this is by finding a constant stream of recipes and ideas that can be incorporated into your diet to avoid the boredom of repetition. Ensure that your source of information is Ketogenic friendly. Educate yourself and beware of all the self styled experts on the web doling out advice.

# Chapter 6: What to Eat

It is good that you are interested in trying out the Ketogenic diet. But when you have got no idea about the food products that you should and shouldn't consume, following a diet would be an absolute nightmare. In this chapter, provided is a comprehensive list of the things that you can and cannot eat. Being conscious of what you eat is the first step of ensuring that the diet is going to be effective. If you are suffering from any condition that causes imbalances in the levels of blood sugar in your body, consult your doctor before starting the diet.

Read through this chapter carefully.

## Fats and oils

The major portion of your calorie intake will come from this category on a daily basis. Fats are essential for the functioning of your body but these can prove to be incredibly dangerous when the wrong types of fat are consumed. Balance out Omega 3 and Omega 6 fatty foods. Trout, salmon, tuna and even shellfish can help maintain the required balance of Omega 3 in your daily diet. Supplements are recommended to people with allergic reactions to seafood or have a dislike to seafood. Fish oil supplements maintain the required amount of Omega 3 in the body.

For saturated and monounsaturated fats, consume butter, macadamia nuts, egg yolks and avocado as well. These products have chemical stability and don't cause any inflammation. Combine fats and oils together and add this to your meals in different ways. You can make sauces or even dressings for your salads or just add a dollop of butter to your meats. Avoid hydrogenated fats as well as trans fats. Steer clear of products like margarine. Studies show that the consumption of such undesirable fats is directly proportional to the risk of heart diseases. Cold pressed oils are the best choice if you are using vegetable oils such as olive oil, soya bean or even sunflower oil. In frying, make use of non hydrogenated oils like beef tallow, ghee or even coconut oil because the smoke point of these oils is usually high allowing for lesser oxidization. This ensures that your body will receive more of the necessary fatty acids. Also, watch the amount of nuts or any seed based food that you eat. These contain Omega 6 and is inflammatory in nature. Eat almonds, walnuts, pine nuts and even some seed-based oils in moderation.

The following are a great source of both oils and fats that you can include in the diet: avocado, beef tallow, chicken fat, macadamia nuts, butter, ghee, mayonnaise and any other non-hydrogenated lard, coconut oil, olive oil, sunflower oil or even peanut oil. If any of the above mentioned products are available in the organic or the grass fed range, choose those instead of the regular ones.

## Protein

The variety of produce for you to choose from for meeting the daily requirement of protein is quite varied. Whenever possible opt for the organic or grass fed meats as they are healthier. The list of proteins that you can choose from are:

**Fish:** Tuna, flounder, mahi mahi, catfish, cod, salmon, snapper, mackerel, trout, halibut, and anything caught in the wild is a safe bet.

**Shellfish:** Squid, lobster, crabs, scallops, oyster, mussels and clams.

**Eggs:** Get the free range eggs whenever possible. Consume a whole egg and don't discard the yolk. You can scramble, poach, fry, devil or just boil them.

**Meat:** Grass fed meets are a better option compared to the steroid injected meats available these days. Beef, veal, goat, lamb and any other game meat are good choices.

**Pork:** Pork loin, chops and ham are good though watch out for any added sugars when consuming pork.

**Poultry:** Opt for free-range produce whenever you can. Chicken, duck, quail, and pheasant are the recommended.

**Bacon:** Whenever you want to consume bacon and sausages, check the labels thoroughly to see that it does not contain any extra filler and is not cured in sugar.

**Peanut butter:** This can contain Omega 6 and even carbs, so be careful while consuming peanut butter. Other choice is macadamia nut butter.

## Vegetables

Vegetables are essential. While following the Ketogenic diet, choose vegetables that are grown above ground like leafy green vegetables. Organic vegetables have additional nutrients when compared to non-organic produce. Some vegetables just don't meet the nutritional cut for this diet. The best type of vegetables need to keep in tune with the basic principle of the Keto diet: they should be low carb. Yes, you guessed it right, dark and leafy vegetables are the best options. Spinach or even kale can be consumed without any second thoughts. The vegetables that you can eat while in keto diet include: avocado, asparagus, broccoli, cauliflower, carrots, celery, green beans, cucumber, garlic, mushrooms, green onions, bell peppers, pickles, dill, romaine lettuce, shallots, snow peas, squash, spinach, kale and tomatoes. Avoid potatoes, sweet potatoes among others.

## Dairy Products

Dairy products are an essential part of your diet. Choose the full fat produce. If you can get your hands on raw and organic milk products, you can consume heavy whipping cream, hard and soft cheeses, sour cream and milk. Cheese lovers needn't give up on their love for cheese but don't overeat. Dairy products address your fat and calcium requirements.

## Nuts and seeds

Nuts are probably the best way to get rid of all the anti-nutrients present. Do avoid peanuts, since they fall under the category of legumes and legumes are not a part of the Ketogenic diet. Nuts are really good for the health but this does not give you the reason to overeat. You can have almonds, walnuts and macadamia nuts in small quantities. Cashews and pistachios contain more carbs than previously mentioned nuts. Nuts have a high content of Omega 6, so eat in moderate quantities. Instead of regular flour, choose flour made out of nuts and seeds like almond flour and flax seed flour. This gives you the freedom to indulge yourself in guilty pleasures every once in a while while steering clear of the regular flour.

## Beverages

Ensure that you are fully hydrated while following the Ketogenic diet because it is diuretic in nature. Be more cautious if you are susceptible to urinary tract infection or bladder pain as well. Keep your body hydrated throughout the day. Drink at least 8 glasses of water and a little more if you can manage to. Keep drinking liquids but avoid anything that has artificial sweeteners, fruit juices or any packaged drinks. Coffee and tea can also be consumed in moderation with very little sugar as much as possible. Stay away from soda and other aerated drinks.

# Chapter 7: Five Common Low-carb Mistakes

In this chapter, we will take a look at five rookie mistakes that are committed while dieting and the ways you can avoid them. If you really want your body to enter ketosis in its true sense, then just cutting back on carbs won't do the trick. If you haven't gotten the optimal results after following the Ketogenic diet, then it is more than likely that you have been committing the following mistakes.

## Consumption of carbs

There is no proper definition of the term "low-carb." This changes from person to person and even the region they live in. For instance, anything below 100 and 150 grams per day will be considered low in carbs according to the Western standards. A lot of people might even be able to achieve the optimal results even after consuming the above mentioned amount of carbs provided they stayed away from processed foods. Generally, if you keep the consumption of carbs below 50 grams per day, it will help your body to enter ketosis. If you really want your body to enter the full ketosis mode, then even this amount of carbs is undesirable. Experimentation with your diet is the best way to figure out the amount of carbs that you can consume. This means that the sources of carbs become limited and you will have to choose from vegetables and small quantities of fruits.

To make the most of this diet then it is recommended that you limit your carb consumption to less than 50 grams per day.

## Consumption of protein

Protein is the main source of energy in this diet. It makes you feel full, reduces your appetite in a good way and it also increases the ability of your body to burn out fat when compared to other micronutrients. To put it simply, the consumption of more protein will help in rapid weight loss. In a low-carb diet, you will still need to mind the amount of protein you are consuming. Eating more protein than what is required by the body will convert amino acids to glucose. Once this happens, your body cannot go into full ketosis. A proper Ketogenic diet should be low in the content of carbohydrates, high in fat and should include moderate amount of proteins. The suitable range for consumption of protein would be anywhere between 1.5 and 2 grams per kilo. Avoid gluconeogenesis, the process of conversion of protein into glucose, and try to keep your consumption of protein within the desired ranges.

## Shying away from fat

Most of the calories we consume come from carbs specifically from sugars and various grains. When you stop consuming carbohydrates, a substitute source of energy is necessary. Assuming that low-carb diet goes in hand with low fat diet is a bad idea. The Ketogenic diet restricts the carbs to be replaced with healthy fats. There is no reason to be scared of consuming fats as long as you opt for good fats like Omega 3's and saturated fats.

## Replacement of sodium

The mechanism at work that makes the Ketogenic diet a success is the reduction in the level of insulin that is produced in the body. Insulin is essential for your body because it helps the cells balance glucose, to store fat and signals the kidneys to keep some sodium in the body. In Ketogenic diet, the amount of insulin generated in the body gets reduced wherein the body starts getting rid of sodium along with water. This is why people tend to shed a few kilos within days of following the Keto diet. It is really important that your body has sufficient sodium because it is an electrolyte. One of the main reasons for the failure of this diet would be the reduction in the sodium content present in the body. Its side effects are fatigue, frequent headaches, constipation and even lightheadedness. The best way to avoid this is to add sodium to your diet. Add a little bit of salt to your food. Another way to address this is to consume a cup of broth. You can make a meal out of it as well. Make some light broth, add some lean protein or vegetables and there you have it, a healthy soup.

When you reduce the consumption of carbs, insulin produced is reduced as well. This means the body starts getting rid of sodium as well and might cause a mild deficiency of sodium.

## Show some patience

The body is naturally gives preference to burn carbs provided they are available. When you get rid of carbs in your diet, the body will move towards burning fat to generate energy. This adaptation is going to take a few days and during this stage of initiation you might feel a little out of sorts. This is natural and referred to as the low-carb flu. The time taken by your body to fully adapt itself to the burning of fat molecules for the production of energy can take a few weeks. So, be patient and stick to your diet. Let the metabolism of your body get used to this diet. The results generated will be nothing short of miraculous.

# Chapter 8: Science Behind the Ketogenic Diet

When it comes to the ketogenic diet, there are some things that work in its favor. This means that the diet will have a positive bearing on your body, which will aid in you losing your excess weight.

## Protein intake

The body needs proteins for many purposes. When you consume excess proteins, you end up increasing the metabolic activity in your body. This in turn causes your body to remain slim for long. Proteins are very filling. They will help you feel full without having to eat too much. You will also feel energetic and not feel the need to consume any sugar.

## Water break down

Have you heard of water weight? It refers to the weight of the water inside the body. Fat in the body generally stores some water. Once that is freed, the body weight will automatically come down. In the ketogenic diet, your body will start shedding the excess water from the body. The water will also take away with it toxins which will further add to your body's health.

## General metabolism

The ketogenic diet helps in setting the body's metabolism in motion. It aids in accelerating the body metabolism and you will feel stronger and fitter within a few days of being on the diet. You might feel lighter as well because the food will not stay in your body for too long. Hence, the ketogenic diet will help you remain stronger and fitter for a long time.

# Chapter 9: Mistakes to Avoid with the Diet

## Not planning ahead

Without a concrete plan in place will cause you to not take the diet seriously. Create a plan of action and follow through in order to make the diet a lifetime choice. Imagine what would happen if you went to a foreign country without a map. You would get lost and would not enjoy the journey. Similarly, you should plan out your diet and follow through with it. It does not have to be a military level plan; it can be simple yet effective.

## Calorie intake

Many people make the mistake of not checking whether they are consuming too many calories in a bid to cut down on the carbs. This ends up causing them to go back on their diet's effects on the body. For this, you have to identify the different foods that are full of calories and cut down on them. If you don't know what they are, consider making a list of all the foods that you consume now and then go through each one's calorie content. Surely you will find a few that are highly calorific. Avoid consuming those as much as possible.

## Zero nutrition

Another mistake is eating low carb foods and ending up cutting out all the nutrition as well. This is not the right way to go about in any diet. The nutritional content in the food must be quite high with vitamins, minerals and other nutrients to help the body remain strong. This is possible through a list of all the healthy foods to consume and then try to incorporate them as much as possible in your diet. Once you come up with a meal plan, you will find it easy to see what you are consuming and what extra needs to be added in.

## Fibrous meals

Fiber is an important part of the diet. Consume as much of it as possible in order to aid in digestion. It is ideal for you to increase its intake if you think you're not consuming enough fiber. Some sources of fiber include vegetables, fruits, nuts and seeds. You can munch on these after a meal and help your body digest food better. You will also feel quite energetic and not have to deal with mood swings.

## Munching nuts

It is a great idea for people to munch on nuts, as they are full of essential oils that are great for the body and will keep the joints lubricated. But, it is completely wrong for a person on a low carb diet to consume it as these nuts might cause unnecessary weight gain. It is best for you to avoid consuming them and look at other things as snacking choices. You can, for example, consume cut vegetables such as carrots or beets as they will be sweet and tasty and yet great for your diet.

## Not timing it

It is important to time the consumption of carbohydrates. Although you cannot completely eliminate them from your diet, you can time it right to help digest and get it eliminated better. It is best to consume the carbs just before exercising. The body will get a jump-start and will be able to digest the carbs much easily.

## No supplements

Many people don't realize that it is important to consume supplements in order to maintain a healthy body. These supplements are full of nutrients that will make the body strong and are also going to help you with your diet. You can take some general supplements such as calcium and vitamin tablets to supplement your diet but you might need more. To know what supplements to consume, visit your doctor and seek advice on what supplements you need. Based on your food habits, he or she will suggest the supplements that you should be consuming.

# Being stressed

A lot of unnecessary stress and tension will impact your body negatively. Your mind will make it difficult for you to concentrate on anything, let alone your diet. So it will be quite necessary for you to stop stressing out and relax your mind. Find activities that you can do on a regular basis and reduce your stress levels. You might also have to find out what is causing the stress in the first place and reduce it as much as possible.

# Sleeping less

Sleeping less than your normal sleeping hours can also impact your body negatively. It is impossible to be healthy if you stay up late and not get enough sleep. It is best to get at least 8 hours of sleep and without too many disturbances. Make use of some light music to fall asleep or burn a few aroma candles to help you sleep better. You might also have to drain away as much stress and tension before sleeping in order to avail peaceful sleep.

# Expecting too much

Expecting too much from your diet is never going to help you. Set reasonable expectations and do not go overboard with what you wish to attain from it. Try to go about it one step at a time. Don't start with the diet the previous day and expect to see positive results the next day. It will take a little time but you will see results for sure. Don't worry if you have gone back a little on the diet. You can always catch up and make the most of it once you take it up seriously.

# Too many cheat meals

It is known that the low carb diet allows one cheat meal. These cheat meals are meant to help you stick with the diet. You can have one, once in a while. But, it is important to not get carried away and have too many cheat meals. Some people end up having more than 1 cheat meal a week and simply increase their calorie intake. This might cause you to fall back to your old eating habits. Control yourself as much as possible and set a limit to your cheat meals.

## Not exercising

Exercise is a part of any healthy diet. It helps the body lose some of the excess weight and also cut down on the fat cells. If you don't exercise, then you might not be able to lose weight as fast as you can. Sketch out a weight loss plan and follow through it. The exercises don't have to be too rigorous. We will look at a simple exercise plan at the end of this book that will help you come up with your own exercise and weight loss plan.

These are the mistakes to avoid with the low carb diet.

# Chapter 10: Some drawbacks and their remedies

There are some drawbacks of the ketogenic diet that you should be aware of before taking it up. These drawbacks are quite normal and will not stay too long.

## Frequent urination

When on the low carb or the ketogenic diet, you will feel like urinating too often. This is very common and nothing that you should worry too much about. The diet causes your body to break down the glucose present in your kidney and liver, which might cause a lot of water to release in the body. You have to be prepared to run to the bathroom more often as a result. However, don't assume that drinking less water will help you resolve the issue. There is no correlation between the two and you might not be able to solve the problem. So, don't cut down on the number of glasses of water you gulp down in a day. You should maintain the same, especially if you want the water to further help with your diet.

## Bad breath

Bad breath is another major side effect of the ketogenic diet. Many people complain that their breath has worsened and despite brushing their teeth regularly it still smells quite bad. This is mainly because of ketosis. Although this should not be too much of a problem if you brush your teeth thrice and also clean your tongue, you will be able to stave off the bad breath for a long time. You can also consider rinsing your mouth with mouthwash thrice a day. Munching on a few mint or basil leaves will help you maintain fresh breath.

## Mood swings

Mood swings are a common side effect of the ketogenic diet. Many people complain about being too grumpy one minute and then normal the next. All of this will cause you to feel uneasy. Try to control your mood by consuming the right foods. Increasing your water intake and also the fiber content in your food will go a long way in helping you stave off the mood swings. You will also feel happy if you sip on some fruit infused water.

## Tiredness

Tiredness or fatigue is another complaint that many people have when on the ketogenic diet. Although it is quite common for people on the ketogenic diet to feel tired and out of breath, it is not easy to handle. The excess water that is eliminated from the body will carry with it minerals and salts that are essential for the body. This will cause you to weaken. Therefore, it is important to consume supplements that will help in restoring some of these back into your body. You will feel much more energetic and not feel as dizzy. You can also consume a glass of water to which some salt has been added in. This will help in restoring the salt content in your body and reducing the dizziness.

## Headaches

Headaches are a common aspect of the ketogenic diet. This is also mainly caused by the loss of minerals and salts in the body. Some people also complain of having very little energy and possibly flu like symptoms. If you are feeling any of this, then it is obvious that they are caused by the diet. Taking supplements is the best option and also consuming a little extra salt with your diet. In fact, just increasing the water intake will go a long way in helping you restore your energy and reduce the headaches by some margin.

## Low sugar

Low sugar levels are common amongst keto dieters. The body will be going through the process of cutting down on the fat in the body and that will cause the sugar levels to reduce as well. It is important for your body to maintain a steady sugar level, especially if you wish to remain energetic. You might crave sweets and chocolates, which can be quite bad for the diet. Do not give into your cravings. As for the weakness, munch on vegetables. It will add in some mild glucose which will not interfere with your diet. The sugar craving will disappear after a while and it is best that you ignore it until your body settles in with the diet.

## Constipation

Constipation is another major bodily complaint that most people have when they take up the ketogenic diet. The loss of magnesium and also calcium to some extent will cause you to feel constipated. It will feel like the food is not getting digested so you might experience bloating and uneasiness especially during the initial days of the diet when the body is yet to adjust to it. Constipation can also cause stomachache, which will feel quite uneasy. The best solution is to consume lots of fibrous foods. These foods will help in the bowel movement. You can also consume other foods and supplements that act as mild laxatives and ease bowel movement.

## Diarrhea

It is quite interesting to know that some people feel constipated thanks to the ketogenic diet while some others suffer from diarrhea. The intake of too much protein can cause the digestive system to go for a toss. To remedy this issue, you may take some anti-diarrheal that will help with your digestion.

## Cramps

Some people complain of cramps in the body. These can be muscle or other bodily cramps that might cause you to feel uncomfortable. So, it is important for you to restore the lost minerals from your body. The best way is to consume foods that are rich in the minerals. You can also consume more table salt. The cramps might not be limited to your muscles and might extend to your joints as well. Eat some fresh foods and nutrient oils to help with the process.

## Kidney issues

This side effect is not that common but will mostly come about if you consume too much potassium. This can come through potassium supplements. It is important that you ask your physician if you can take the potassium supplement regularly. He will also prescribe the right amount that you have to take. Consuming a lot of water is a great way to deal with this issue.

## Thyroid issues

Some people might also complain about thyroid issues, T3 to be precise. You will have to consult your physician and ask for a remedy that will help you move past it.

## Lack of sleep

Some people complain of lack of sleep when on the ketogenic diet. This might be true owing to the imbalance on insulin and serotonin levels in the brain. The best solution is to increase the serotonin levels in your brain by taking up activities that will help you increase the serotonin levels such as exercising. Try also to avoid eating close to bedtime as that can cause you to lose sleep.

These are some of the common issues that come along with the ketogenic diet. there is no need for alarm. They will subside after a while as the body gets used to it. Instead of complaining about them, it is best to focus on the remedies to ease the symptoms.

# Chapter 11: Related FAQs

## Are ketogenic and other low carb diets the same?

The ketogenic diet is a diet that induces a state of ketosis. Ketosis refers to a situation where the body starts to burn away the fat and reduces the person's body weight. There are other diets such as the Atkin's diet, which is a low carb diet. But it might not provide the same benefits as the ketogenic diet. Both diets will provide different results and you can choose the one that suits your physique.

## Is it bad to lose too much weight at once?

Generally, yes. You should try and lose weight slowly yet steadily. There must be progress with the weight loss. Do not try to lose all of it within a month or two. Have a weight loss plan in place that is practical. Try to lose not more than a few pounds a month. You should lose the weight based on your body type and weight. If you feel dizzy or weak then you should stop with the diet and consult with a physician to see if the problem can be fixed.

## Can vegans take this diet up?

Yes. The low carb diet allows a wide range of foods to be consumed and does not limit it to just meats. You can consume fresh fruits and vegetables and also lentils. You can come up with a low carb vegan diet plan. If you don't know where to start, then you can research online and find an appropriate diet. Modify it as per your taste. The same extends to vegetarians who can make the addition of dairy products into their diet.

## Is it important to consume lots of proteins as per the low carb diet?

Ideally yes. To make up for all the carbohydrates that are not consumed during the diet, it is important that you substitute it with the proteins. Proteins are known to help with weight reduction. It allows in the production of healthy muscles, which is great for the body. Most proteins come from foods that are part of our everyday diet. So all you have to do is increase their quantity and not go out of your way to incorporate it in your diet. Some of these include meats such as chicken, turkey, eggs, chickpeas, etc.

## How much calories should I consume on a daily basis?

Calorie counting is often tricky. You have to know what each and every ingredient is in your meal and how many calories they carry. It can get a bit too tedious for you and you might give up on it altogether. However, it is best to have a rough idea of each meal and not get too serious about it. Calorie counting is a must no doubt but it is best if you have a rough estimate of how much you are consuming. Ideally, it is advisable to consume between 1500 and 1800 for women and between 1800 and 2200 for men. That will help you with your weight loss process as well.

## Can I continue it for a lifetime?

Yes. It is a great idea for you to continue with the diet for a long time, possibly a lifetime. If you have the capacity to come up with timely meal plans that are easy to prepare then you will find it easy to settle in with the diet. You have to keep yourself motivated and keep aiming higher. There is nothing like being too fit and the more effort you put in, the better the results.

## Are occasional drinks allowed?

Yes, occasional drinks are allowed provided they are low carb and not more than just a small glass. It is best to limit it to just a single drink per month and not any more. Speak with your family and friends. Tell them about your diet and that you will not be consuming any of the drinks that are prohibited as per the diet.

## Are cheat meals allowed?

Yes. In fact, a cheat meal might be a must, as it will keep you motivated. You can use it as a reward and have it once in a while. The meal does not have to be a grand affair. It can be a simple burger or a pizza.

# Chapter 12: Basic Exercise Plans

When it comes to your diet and exercise plan, it is important to follow a set sequence. Here are some of the exercises that you can take up.

## Warm up

Warm up before taking up an exercise routine to avoid injuries. Warming up helps in preparing your body to take up the different exercises without feeling too tired. It is also important to not exercise with a cold body, as the heat will further help you burn fat. The warm up can be quite simple and yet very effective. The warm up routine may consist of a little running or jogging. If you wish to do something less, then you can jog on the spot or run on the treadmill for some time. You can also do something like stand and do a few jumping jacks. As long as your body heats up, it will work well for you.

## Cardio exercises

### Skipping

Skipping is a great activity that you can take up and quite easy as well. You can buy yourself a skipping rope and start skipping. Another way is to hold an imaginary skipping rope in your hand and start skipping. You can alternate between skipping and jumping jacks. Keep a count of your reps so that you don't over exercise or under exercise. You can also make use of a timer to keep time. How much you skip is up to you and you can choose the time or the count based on your capacity. Remember to do more first.

### Jogging

Jogging is the next exercise that you can take up. Jogging is easy to take up and also quite effective. With jogging, all you have to do is find a walkway that is long enough and start taking small jumping steps. Don't mistake jogging with running, as the two are quite different. You can jog for around 30 minutes and then take a little rest. Start jogging again and then rest again. Such interval training will surely help your body feel a good burn. It is also best for all those that are unable to run.

## Running

Running is great for anyone. In fact, you will see maximum weight loss when you run. It is best for you to pick morning time and start running early. You can do about 30 minutes to an hour. This will help with your weight loss. You can find a long walk way or can also run around in a circular motion. One good technique is to run for a minute and then jog for a minute. Run again and jog again. This will help your body get more in less time. Running is also ideal for those who wish to lose weight from their hip and lower abdomen. Running uphill will help with lower abdomen fat and running downhill helps with hip fat. You can run up and down a hill a few times.

## Swimming

Swimming is not only easy to perform but also most effective when it comes to burning and eliminating fat from the body. You can hit the swimming pool 4 to 5 times a week and swim at least 20 laps. You can also do some running motion in the water as that will also help in weight loss. But you have to be serious about exercising and not simply pass your time at the pool.

## Sports

Indulge in sports activities you like. Playing sports is quite fun. You can join your children or find a group you can play sports with. Sports activities get your heart rate up and will also help you feel relaxed. It can be anything like basketball or football or even baseball. As long as you run or jump around, your body will feel the burn. It is best for you to play sports at least 4 times a week.

Apart from these, you can engage in any other cardio exercise that you deem to be effective. It does not have to be picked from a particular list alone. If you think there is something else that will help you and your body, then do so.

# Weight training

It might be important for you to weight train. Weight training involves lifting heavy weights. This is done to train your muscles and make your body more muscular. Weight training is pretty simple to undertake and it is important that you choose the right weights. For women, 5 lbs. is ideal while for men, its 10 lbs. You can increase the weights as you go. Some basic weight training exercises will suffice and you won't have to do too much. Just lifting your forearm up and down will do the trick. Try also the above the shoulder exercises as it will work on both the biceps and triceps. It is best to do weight training after some cardio, as that is when the body will feel the most burn. You can train with weights for 15 to 30 minutes or more if your body has the capacity for it.

## *Chin ups/ push ups*

Chin-ups refer to holding a rod and pulling yourself up against your body weight. This will help you with your biceps and triceps. Hold your hands a little apart from each other. Lift yourself up and try to touch the rod using your chin. This is easier said than done and you should make use of the right technique to complete the motion. Push-ups are the opposite of chin-ups. You will have to place your palms on the floor in front of you. Now lift yourself up and lower your body down using just your arms. This is great for all those that wish to work on their obliques.

## *Resistance Crunches*

Resistance crunches work much better than regular crunches, as they will cause you to put in a bit more effort. Here, you will place some weights on your abdomen or back when you perform the crunches. This will make it a bit difficult for you to perform the crunches. You can ask someone to place the weights on your body while you perform the crunches. Exercise a little precaution while performing the crunches to avoid any unnecessary injury.

## Yoga/ tai chi

Yoga and tai chi poses are not body intensive yet will help in reducing your weight. Here are some poses that you can try.

## Triangle pose

The triangle pose is quite easy to perform and great for your entire body. Start by standing straight with your hands by your side. Now spread your legs a little and bend down to your right side. Place your left palm next to your right foot and try not to bend your legs. Draw in a deep breath while bending down. Hold the pose for a couple of seconds and then raise your body up. Now bend to the other side. You can continue with this for the next 2 to 5 minutes.

## Breathing exercises

Breathing exercises are great for you. Start by sitting on the floor and folding your legs. Now, draw in deep breaths. Focus on your breath and ensure that your exhaled breath is slightly more paced as compared to your inhaled breath. You should literally feel your lower stomach move in and out. Alternately, you can try out Anulom Vilom where you alternate your nostrils to draw in and exhale breath. Both will help you reduce the fat in your stomach or at least loosen it to some extent.

## Bridge pose

The bridge pose is for your back muscles. Start by lying on your back. Now bend your knees such that they point to the sky. Use your palms to bring your heels close to your butt. Now raise your lower back and support your upper body with your shoulders. You can place your hands under your back and interlock your fingers. Hold the pose for a while and then lower yourself down. Repeat the same again.

## Tree pose

Tree pose is easy to perform. Stand straight with your hands by your side. Then lift your feet up using your hands and place it on the inner side of your thigh. Maintain your balance and lift your hands up in the air to make a Namaste above your head. Hold the pose for a few seconds and then lower your hands back down. Now repeat it with the other foot.

## *Bow pose*

Bow pose helps with abs and lower back fat. Lie flat on the ground. Lift up your upper body and also your lower body simultaneously. Now hold your ankles using your palms and pull them in towards your butt. You should push your head as back as possible while looking upwards. Maintain the pose for a few seconds and go back to neutral. Assume the same pose again, wait and release. Keep doing this for the next 5 to 10 minutes.

You don't have to always be too rigorous to lose weight. You can make use of a set of simple movement based exercises as well. Take advantage of the Internet to look up more tai chi poses that you can do. These are just a few of the different exercises you can incorporate in your work out plan to remain fit and healthy.

# Chapter 13: Precautions to Observe on the Diet

There are a few precautions that you have to observe when it comes to the ketogenic diet. Here they are:

## Pregnant women

The diet is safe for most people and might also include pregnant women. Still, consulting your doctor first is the best move to do. He might prescribe a diet that will settle in with you and your unborn baby. The keto diet side effects might aggravate the hormonal imbalances and bodily changes during pregnancy and put a stress on the body more. It is best to wait after you had your baby and had settled to the life changes that comes with it before taking on the keto diet. If you have been on the diet while getting pregnant then you might not need to make too many modifications to it. Still, consulting your doctor is a must.

## Post delivery

New mothers have to consult a doctor as the body needs some time to recover. It is best not to rush into it. Also, the doctor might suggest something else to help you get back to your pre-pregnancy body and still remain fit.

## Elders

It is important for elders to consult a doctor as well and know if any modifications are needed to be made in the diet. Get a list of supplements and other things that will help with the diet. The doctor might also modify some of the medications being taken.

## Children

Parents need to exercise a little precaution when it comes to putting their children on the ketogenic diet. Because of their age and special nutritional needs, their diets might have to be modified a bit. You can work closely with a dietician to come up with a diet plan. If your child is quite fat, plan an exercise routine along with the diet plan to help avail dual benefits.

## Illness

If you already suffer from a condition like diabetes or heart disease, speak with your doctor beforehand for appropriate advice. If you are taking any medications, then you can ask if you can take the medicine along with the diet.

## Supplements

Before you take any of the supplements, it is best that you ask your doctor first. He will tell you if it is safe to consume them. Some supplements might also react with some medicines and so you will have to ask your physician. The dosages will also differ from person to person thus be careful with the dosage.

These are some of the cases where extra precautions are needed. Somehow, they should not deter you from taking up the diet.

# Chapter 14: How to Stick to The Low Carb Diet

When it comes to taking up a new diet, it is obvious that both your body and mind will resist it. Certain measures are needed to make the habit stay. This chapter will look on the steps on how to stick to your diet.

## Do your research

The first and foremost advice is to do as much research on the topic as possible. Research will help you know what the diet is and how you can go about it. This book will give you a lot of information on the diet and how to go about it no doubt. Still, do not limit yourself to just the information present in this book. It is important that you look outside it as well. You will have to look for websites that will give you valuable and reliable information on the topic and also increase its worth. You can also turn to some publications for the same. A little research and understanding will go a long way towards helping you turn it into a lifetime habit.

## Create a time table

A timetable will come in handy and help you carry out your diet easily. The timetable can be simple with the different activities and the respective timings mentioned next to it. You can make two columns where the first one mentions the activity and the other column the time. The activities can be like eat a snack, exercise etc. Anything that helps you stick with the diet will cause you to remain with it for a long time.

## Maintain a record

Many people find it extremely motivating to maintain a record of their experiences. They prefer to maintain a journal and write down their daily experiences with the diet. This can include the effects that the diet have on the body, weight loss, higher energy levels, etc. You will see your progress better and that your body is getting fitter. It will motivate you to continue with the diet for long and not stop with it. You can either maintain a physical journal or a digital one. A digital one will be easy to maintain and also refer back.

## Find a partner

A partner will not only help you remain motivated to continue with the diet but also make it easier for you. You will not have to prepare different meals for the different members of your family. If all of them are following the diet with you, then the meals will be quite easy to prepare. If your spouse is also following the diet, then he or she might help you stay on course. But it need not always be a spouse, a friend or a sibling can be your partner as well.

## Find a group

Just like a partner, you can also choose to join a group. The group can be a ketogenic diet group that meets up in your area to discuss the effects of the diet and also other aspects of it. If the group is not present in your area, then you can create one yourself. Just ask your friends if they are interested in it or already follow the diet. Then invite them over and discuss the diet in detail with them. That will surely help you remain with the diet for long.

## Prepare meal plans

Meal plans are a great way to feel motivated to follow the ketogenic diet. You can create the meal plans well in advance and follow them through. We've included some basic meal plans that you can follow and also some recipes that you can try out. These will surely give you a head start. You can also consider cleaning up your kitchen by disposing off the fatty and sugary foods and stacking up on the healthy and keto friendly foods. This will help you remain motivated.

## Appreciate your body

Those who love their body and remain appreciative of it will find it rather easy to maintain a diet. They will not take it for granted and put in necessary efforts to maintain a slim and trim body. The same will extend to you if you wish to make full use of the ketogenic diet. You have to appreciate your body to keep it healthy. Take some time out to go through your diet once in a while and see if it is helping you remain fit and healthy.

## Reward yourself

Nothing works better than rewarding yourself with something nice from time to time. This need not be a food reward. Although many people would consider the celebration meal to be a reward in itself, you might have to do much more. This can include visiting a spa for a relaxing massage, taking a vacation, buying yourself something nice, etc. All of it will go a long way in helping you remain in the diet. But make sure you don't reward yourself too often and to leave a little gap between one reward and the next.

## Speak about it

It is a good idea for you to speak about the diet to as many people as possible. You can also profess about it as that will motivate your further. You can try speaking about it on an online site or blog about it. You can also post pictures of yourself from before and after. That will help you remain motivated and continue with the diet for a long time. However, you must prepare to read a few nasty comments about the diet. They might seem harsh. Learn to ignore them and focus on the positive ones.

These are just some of the things that you can do to remain motivated with the diet. Do not be limited to just these. Be creative and do whatever it takes to stick with your diet.

# Chapter 15: Sumptuous Recipes

## Breakfast recipes

### *Cheddar omelet with fresh salad*
Ingredients:
- 3 large eggs, slightly beaten
- 1 tablespoon mixed herbs, parsley, basil, cilantro, chopped
- Salt to taste
- Black pepper to taste
- 1 tablespoon unsalted butter
- 2 tablespoons fresh goat cheese

Recipe:
Place the griddle on heat. Combine the eggs, herbs (reserve some for the cheese), salt and pepper in a bowl and whisk until well combined. Add the butter to the pan and allow it to melt. Put the beaten eggs to make an omelet. While the egg is cooking, place the cheese in a bowl and crumble it along with the herbs and mix well. Open the omelet on a plate and sprinkle the goat's cheese. Fold the omelet and serve hot.

### *Chicken and mushroom breakfast*
Ingredients:
- 4 small eggs
- 2 chicken Breast, skinned
- 3 tablespoons scallions, chopped
- 2 tablespoons Olive Oil
- 1 cup mushrooms, chopped
- Salt to taste
- Black pepper to taste
- Italian seasoning, to taste
- 1/4 cup shredded Mozzarella Cheese

Recipe:

Beat the eggs in a bowl along with the salt, pepper and seasoning and mix until well combined. Cut the chicken breasts into small pieces and add it to the egg mix. Meanwhile, add the oil to the pan and allow it to heat. Sauté the chopped scallions. Add in the mushrooms and the marinated chicken. Sauté until the chicken is soft. Remove from pan, sprinkle the mozzarella on top and serve hot.

# Lunch recipes

### Stuffed bottle gourd
Ingredients:
- 1 large bottle gourd
- 1 large red onion, chopped
- 1 large tomato, chopped
- 2 tablespoons garlic
- ½ inch ginger stick, peeled and grated
- 1 tablespoon oil
- Salt to taste
- Pepper to taste
- ¼ the cup mozzarella cheese

Recipe:

Heat oil and sauté chopped onions and garlic in a pan. Once it browns, add in the tomato, salt and pepper. Give it a good mix. Meanwhile, preheat the oven to 350 degrees Fahrenheit. Cut the top of the bottle gourd and cut it into 3 to 4 cylinders. Use a spoon to scoop out the centers of the gourd and add it to the tomato mix. Place the cylinders on a baking tray. Fill each of them with the tomato mix and sprinkle the cheese on top.

Place it in the oven for 20 to 30 minutes. Serve hot.

### Chickpea salad
Ingredients:
- 1 cup chickpeas, boiled

- 1 large tomato
- 1 red onion
- 1 zucchini
- 1 tablespoon olive oil
- 1 tablespoon mustard
- Salt to taste
- Pepper to taste

Recipe:
Chop the tomatoes, onion and zucchini into small pieces. Add the mustard and oil to a small bowl and mix until well combined. Add the chickpeas to a bowl along with the chopped vegetables. Now add the salt and pepper and mix until well combined.
Add in the mustard and oil paste and serve.

# Dinner recipes

## *Shrimpy devilled eggs*
Ingredients:
- 4 large Boiled Eggs
- 2 tablespoons low fat mayonnaise, homemade or store bought
- 2 tablespoons pickles
- 1/2 teaspoon mustard
- 1/2 teaspoon horseradish (optional)
- 1/8 teaspoon pepper sauce
- 8 fresh larges shrimps
- Salt to taste
- Cilantro to sprinkle

Recipe:
Cut the eggs into half and scoop out the yellow from the center. Put it in a bowl along with the mayonnaise, pickle, horseradish, mustard, pepper sauce and salt. Mix well. Now spoon a teaspoon or so of the yolk mix inside the egg halves. Place one shrimp each on top of each of the yolk. You can press it in a little to help it stay in place. Sprinkle some of the cilantro on top and serve.

## Turkey sausages

Ingredients:

- 2 tablespoons onions, chopped
- 1 cup turkey Sausages, cut into pieces
- 1 tablespoon oil
- Salt to taste
- Pepper to taste
- 1/3 cup chopped green pepper
- 2 tablespoons mozzarella cheese

Recipe:

Heat the oil in a pan. Add in the chopped onion. Allow it to sauté for a while or until it browns. Then add in the green pepper along with the salt and pepper and give it a good mix. Add in the sausages and sauté it until it browns and softens. Sprinkle the cheese on top and serve hot.

# Ketogenic drink recipes

## Simple lemon tea

Ingredients:

- 1 teaspoon regular tea powder
- 1 lemon
- 1 cup water
- ½ teaspoon honey, optional

Recipe:

Heat water in a pan. Add the tea powder and allow it to boil. Then strain it into a cup. Squeeze in the lemon and mix well. Add in the honey, stir and serve hot. This can also be cooled and served as cold tea.

## Cleansing drink

Ingredients:

- 1 cup kale, chopped
- ½ cup green peppers, chopped

- 1 zucchini
- Salt
- Coconut milk as needed

Recipe:
Add all the ingredients to a blender and make a smooth puree. Add in as much coconut milk as needed and serve.

## Easy juice pops
Ingredients:
- 1 cup melon pieces
- 1 cup papaya pieces
- 1 cup strawberries
- 1 cup blueberries
- ½ cup lemon juice
- ½ cup fresh mint leaves, chopped

Recipe:
Put all the fruits in a juicer and make a fresh juice. Add in the lemon juice and mix well. Pour the juice into Popsicle molds. Drop in a few mint leaves into each and freeze.

## Black tea infuse
Ingredients:
- 2 black tea bags
- 2 cups water
- 1 cup rose petals
- Honey to taste (optional)

Recipe:
Boil water in a pan. Add in the rose petals and allow it to infuse. Put the tea bags in a cup. Add in the rose infused water and allow the tea bag to steep for a while. Serve it hot.

## Green tea with fruits

Ingredients:

- 2 green tea bags
- 2 cups water
- ½ cup apples, chopped
- ½ cup grapes, whole
- ½ cup melon, chopped
- Hone to taste

Recipe:

Boil water in a pan. Put the tea bags in a cup and pour the hot water. Put cut fruits in a bowl and add the honey. Mix well. Pour the tea on top and mix. Serve cold.

## Coconut surprise

Ingredients:

- 1 cup coconut water
- ½ cup coconut cream
- ½ cup pineapple, chopped
- Honey to taste
- Mint leaves to sprinkle.

Recipe:

Put the coconut cream and pineapple pieces in a blender and whizz until smooth. Add the honey and coconut water and whizz again until well blended. Add in some crushed ice to the mix. Serve cold with a few mint leaves sprinkled on top.

# Chapter 16: Shopping List to Carry with you / 1 Week Ketogenic Diet Plan

## Aisles to avoid

- Processed, refined sugars: soft drinks, store bought juices, agave, candies, ice creams and other processed foods that contain sugar.
- Gluten Grains: Wheat, oats, rye, barley and all foods made from these.
- Trans Fats: Anything marked as hydrogenated or poly hydrogenated.
- High-level Omega-6 oils and Vegetable Oils: sunflower, safflower, pomace, cottonseed oil, soya bean oil, etc.
- Artificial Sweeteners: None of the ready available brands are allowed for consumption. Sauces and condiments.
- Any products that carry diet or low fat markings. They all might contain unnecessary chemicals.
- Any other processed foods that you think are not right for you or your diet. Avoid consuming any unnecessary readymade foods.

## Shopping list to carry with you

- Meat: chicken, lamb, beef, pork and other grass fed meat
- Fish: bass, trout, salmon and other wild fish
- Eggs: Free-range eggs
- Vegetables: Broccoli, Spinach, carrots, cauliflower, and many others
- Fruits: kiwis, pineapples, apples, papaya, watermelon, blueberries, strawberries, etc.
- Nuts - Seeds: walnuts, pine nuts, hazel nuts, cashew nuts, and almonds
- High-Fat Dairy: yogurt, cheese, cream, butter, ghee

- Fats and Oils: olive oil, coconut oil, almond oil, cashew oil, and groundnut oil

## Monday

Breakfast: Omelet with goat's cheese (recipe included in this book)
Lunch: Low fat fresh yogurt with strawberries and a few cashews roasted and slivered (make sure the fat from it does not escape while roasting)
Dinner: simple vegetable salad dressed with cold fresh low fat yogurt

## Tuesday

Breakfast: chicken and mushroom breakfast (recipe included in this book)
Lunch: Any leftover fresh vegetable salad with cold fresh yogurt, you can add in some fresh vegetables if you like.
Dinner: sautéed vegetables with grilled chicken and hot sauce

## Wednesday

Breakfast: egg frittata with colorful vegetables
Lunch: baked salmon with some olive oil and garlic drizzle
Dinner: fruit salad with a little strawberry yogurt

## Thursday

Breakfast: left over fruit salad with strawberry yogurt, add in some fresh fruits to it
Lunch: cleansing smoothie with kale, pepper, MCT oil and cucumbers
Dinner: chicken patties with roasted vegetables

## Friday

Breakfast: omelets with crispy bacon
Lunch: shrimp cocktail with low fat yogurt sauce
Dinner: beef stew

## Saturday

Breakfast: devilled eggs with avocado
Lunch: pork ribs roasted and salsa sauce

Dinner: mixed vegetable salad with fresh yogurt

## Sunday

Breakfast: left over mixed vegetable salad with fresh yogurt, add in some fresh vegetables
Lunch: spicy chicken breasts with cauliflower rice
Dinner: one cheat meal, 1 small burger with ideally whole-wheat bun

This is a good meal plan to start with to help you get started with the diet at the earliest.

# Chapter 17: Things You Will Need While On the Diet

When it comes to losing weight and body fat, it is best that you do everything in your power to see results. In this chapter, we will look at some of the things that you may need to continue with the diet for a long time.

## Weighing machine

You have to buy yourself a weighing machine. It is probably the most important thing that you will need for your journey. Many people argue that a person's weight does not really tell whether he or she is fat. There is water weight and also bone density to account for. However, it will give an accurate measure of your real weight. It will tell you how heavy you really are and how much weight you should have. You can either buy a digital one or a conventional machine. The former will give you an accurate measure.

## Pressure cooker

Buying a pressure cooker for yourself will prove to be a big boon. You will find it quite easy to cook your meals without having to put in too much effort. All you do is put in all the ingredients, add water and allow it to blow 3 to 5 whistles. Wait for the steam to escape and your meal will be ready. It will be a one-pot solution that will surely help you cook the meals fast.

## Instant pot

You can also buy yourself an instant pot. It is a pressure cooker, a slow cooker and a steamer all in one. This generally run on electricity and will help you cook with ease. It also have an instant steam release vent that will help release the steam fast. It is also good to reheat food. A slow cooker will help you cook the food slowly and help preserve most of the nutrition in the food. All you have to do is put the food into the instant pot and the food will be hot and ready in no time at all.

## Body fat machine

A body fat machine is different from a weighing machine. It is one that will help measure the fat in your body. A person might appear slim but the fat content in the body might be more. So, you will have to buy a body fat percentage monitor to see how much fat is present in your body. The limit differs from person to person but in general it is limited to 6% per person. You can know the exact values by doing a quick Internet search.

## Tea infuser

We looked at some easy tea recipes that you can try out. They will help you beat your hunger pangs and also cleanse your body from the inside. You can buy a tea infuser to help you prepare the tea with ease. All you have to do is add in some powder or leaves in one section and some hot water in the other and your tea will be infused. You don't have to worry about heating water or finding a strainer. You can simply strain the tea into a cup with much ease.

## Air fryer

The latest technology in the world of health care is an air fryer. The air fryer is one where you will not need to use too much oil to prepare food. You will only have to apply a little by making use of a brush. You won't have to bust out the deep fryer and your fritters and other such food items will be ready within no time. This is great for people looking to eat their favorite foods without the added carbs or calories.

## Miscellaneous

Apart from these, you can also buy some other things that you think will help you with your weight loss journey. You can buy a few ketogenic recipe books if you like or also a ketogenic food chart. These will help you stay on course.

# Key highlights

First and foremost, it is important to understand what the ketogenic diet is all about. If you don't know what it means or stands for and simply decide to take it up, then it will not work for you. Put in efforts to do as much research on the topic as possible.

As you know by now, the keto diet is a low carb diet. Low carb refers to low carbohydrates that are to be consumed by the dieter. Carbohydrates give people the sugar or energy to survive. But too much of it will cause it to be converted to fat. So, by consuming less carbohydrates and increasing the protein intake, you will successfully burn the fat in the body. Therefore, these diets are great for all those that wish to attain a slim body.

The next thing is to plan out your diet. It is important to have a set plan. Do not randomly start on it and expect to see results. Have a schedule in place. Start by weighing yourself and then deciding on how much you plan to lose. Based on it you can come up with the ketogenic plan. The main aim of the plan is to cut down on the consumption of carbohydrates. Schedule it either for more than a week or a month. It is important to plan it out in a way that you can stick with it from start to finish. Be inspired by other people who have taken up the diet. You can try asking them and coming up with a plan for yourself. But don't copy the plan as is. It should cater to your body type and must not be generic in nature. The plan should be such that it helps you with your weight loss mission and is not a fancy timetable for you.

There are some mistakes to watch out for when you are on the diet. These mistakes might cause you to go back to your old eating patterns and habits and might reduce its effectivity on your body.

The ketogenic diet comes with a few common side effects. They are a part and parcel of the diet and you will experience some or all of them at some point during your diet. However, precautionary measures are available to counter them. Once your body gets used to the diet, you will not feel like they are big problems at all. Learn to look past them and remain focused on your diet.

We've given some of the best recipes you can try. These recipes are all easy to prepare and will not take too much time. Ensure all the ingredients are ready before hand so that you can reach into the right boxes and cook them for mealtimes. You can also make them in advance and keep them in the fridge. Grab and go meals will surely help you remain fit and healthy.

Some cleaning up will be necessary to stay on course like clearing out your current kitchen or pantry and throwing out all the unnecessary foods, stacking up on foods that are in keeping with the diet, etc. These will help you remain motivated and will do more towards turning it into a habit. Bring a shopping list with all the different foods that are allowed in the diet when you hit the supermarket. You can also buy them online and order from the same list on a monthly basis.

The meal plans that were mentioned in this book are meant to help you get a head start. You can either make use of the same or use it as a blueprint to come up with your own meal plans. They will surely help you prepare the meals with ease and not have to sweat it out. Encourage your family members to take up the diet with you and avail its benefits. It will also be easy for you, as you will only have to prepare one meal and not different ones.

The diet is great for weight loss no doubt but you will have to consume a few supplements in order to help your body remain fit and healthy. Consult with your physician to know which supplements will suit your body. This step is especially important if you are pregnant or nursing or are a senior citizen. These supplements might also react with some medicines that you are already taking and so, it is best that you consult your physician first. Most of these supplements are available over the counter but you might need a prescription for others.

It is extremely important for you to exercise in order to lose weight faster. A healthy diet will not suffice, especially if you plan on losing weight at an elevated pace. Come up with an exercise plan that will help in burning the fat and also get the body to burn away the sugar and carbohydrates. Those who do not exercise and rely only on the diet might see slower results and in some cases, the lost weight is added back on.

There are many things that you can do to stay on the diet. Try and do your best to convert the ketogenic diet into a lifetime choice. Some of the ideas include rewarding yourself, joining a group etc. Do whatever you think will work for you to best stay on course. Once you start seeing the results, you will be motivated to stick with the diet and reel in both health and happiness.

# Conclusion

Thank you once again for choosing this book.

Ketogenic diet is a way of life and all about improving your health by working along with your body and not against it. Experiment with the diet and exercise options available, keep track of your progress and find which works best for you.

Get started right now. It is not that difficult, a little bit of effort can work wonders for you! So get going and all the best!

Thank you!

# Special Invitation!

If you liked what you read and would like to read high quality books, get free bonuses, and get notified first of **FREE EBOOKS,** then join the official Xcension Publishing Company Book Club! Membership is free, but space is limited!
Join the Book Club by visiting the link below:
http://www.xcensionpublishing.com/book-club

# Free Bonus!

As promised, here is your free Low-Carb Cookbook! Just click the visit the link below to download!
http://www.xcensionpublishing.com/LowCarbCookbookBC.pdf

# STOP!

Before you go, kindly do me a HUGE favor and review this book. I would GREATLY appreciate it! Whether you liked the book or not, your feedback is invaluable, as it will be incorporated into later editions to improve this book! You can easily review my book by going back on Amazon.com and viewing your past orders!